Mindful Eating

50 Healthy Habits for a Diet-Free Life

Nancy Popkin

ISBN-13:
978-1986504973

ISBN-10:
1986504972

DEDICATION

To my dear clients: past, present and future.
Our struggles are all the same.

Contents

Introduction

For 12 years I have helped clients from as young as 4 years old to as mature as 92 change their foods and habits to achieve better health. It's a mission that started around the idea of helping people find the right foods for their bodies. And while that is still part of my work, my own personal experience with trauma, post traumatic stress and chronic anxiety led me to realize good health for most of us is not just about what we eat, but also how we eat.

Stress, boredom, fear and exhaustion can lead to bad habits and not taking care of ourselves. That may be stating the obvious. But just how to shift and change habits isn't always easy to identify. We can *try* a restrictive diet that eliminates whatever is keeping us from losing weight, having more energy or feeling good. Unless our thoughts and feelings are part of the program, we will probably not succeed in sticking to it.

I have written this book to share the practices I use with my clients. Some are about "doing" something differently. Others are about thinking about things differently. Some involve food choices; others address cravings and body image or just generally reducing stress - because we know stress leads to less healthy food and beverage choices and over consumption.

Use these practices in the manner that works best for you. Find your favorites that resonate and go back to them again and again. Work through them from 1 to 50 and notice, which stick as new habits. Or just open the book when you need some support and see what you land on.

nancypopkin.com

The Pause

The first practice is the one practice that will help you with most of the other practices. The pause.

For the next several days when you go to reach for the food that contributes extra calories to your diet: the food you nibble on when you are cooking dinner; the food your kids leave on the their plates, or their unfinished snacks; the Girl Scout cookies in freezer; you know the food I'm talking about - whatever is sabotaging you in your most vulnerable moments. – I want you to use the pause.

Set the timer on your phone for 2 minutes and just breathe. Don't eat the food. Don't do anything. Just pause and breathe. See if you can go longer and longer until you don't even want the food any longer. Concentrate on feeling your belly fill up on the inhale and empty on the exhale.

Learning to use the pause will help you stop yourself before doing any kind of damage - whether it's eating unwanted food or firing off a nasty text message. If you don't have your phone timer handy, try counting backwards from 100 to 1.

Use the same pause to disengage from an emotional trigger that would lead to unhealthy eating or any other unhealthy behavior.

Do anything but (stress or boredom) eat

Buy a package of 3x5 cards - On one card, write yourself a pass for x amount of hours, you will use this card once a week, or so, to indulge when you go out with friends or family or attend a social gathering with food.

On all the other cards write one thing you can do other than eat:
- Do your nails
- Read a book
- Write a letter
- Meditate
- Take a bath
- Listen to a podcast for inspiration
- Phone a friend
- Feel your feelings

Fill out as many cards in the pack with non-food activities.

When you are tempted to eat when you are mad, sad, glad, afraid or bored - choose one card and act on what it says. When you are done, if you still want to engage in emotional eating, pick another card.

-3-

Who are your stakeholders?

Make a list of your stakeholders - these are the people in your life who are your supporters. They love you because they are friends or relatives and they want to see you reach your goals. These are people who you will ask to be available to you when you need support around making healthy choices and sticking to healthy habits. This includes support around relationships and other stressors.

Once you have your list of stakeholders, plan how you will ask them to be a stakeholder for you. Will you call them? Send an email explaining your goals and why you need their support? Be sure to let them know how you will reach out to them and how you would like them to respond.

I had a client whose husband was verbally abusive and told her that she couldn't achieve the weight loss her doctor required before performing a surgery she wanted and needed. She texted her stakeholders when she needed encouragement to make good choices and for the strength to disregard his put-downs.

Feel your feelings and inquire

Eating is often a way to avoid feeling our emotions and taking action to change a bad situation.

When we think mad, glad, sad, fear or boredom related thoughts, we are more likely to eat food for the purpose of making us feel better.

We often use food to avoid facing our feeling. I find that once I correctly identify an emotion the uncomfortable feeling that goes with it dissipates fairly quickly.

Instead of reaching for food, feel where that emotion is coming from. For me if I am sad, I often feel it in my heart. If I am fearful, I feel it in my stomach.

After identifying where you feel the emotion in your body, ask yourself some questions about the thoughts related to it, and whether the thoughts are really true. And what the feelings really mean. For instance, if you are sad because you can't be with someone you love, reframe that thought to be happy that you are in that loving relationship. And ask yourself if that relationship would really be changed if you could be together right in this instance, or if you could be together later. Breathe into the spot in your body where you feel the emotion. Inquire some more.

Fear is one of the strongest emotions, and the basis for most destructive behaviors - like staying in bad relationships, bad jobs and bad living situations. When you feel fear, breathe into the place in your body where you feel the fear. Then, question yourself. What are you really afraid of? Being alone? Why? And then question whether those thoughts are really true thoughts. Will you really never be able to support yourself? Will you find another job? Question whatever your fear thoughts are. Ask yourself if the fear is protecting you from something reasonable, or whether it's holding you back from achieving what you want. Sometimes it's both.

What's your story?

We all have an inner dialogue. For some of us the stories we tell ourselves over and over again shape our actions. Whether it's "I will never be thin, so I might as well eat the cookies." Or, whether it is I don't deserve to be happy, so I'll just stay in this relationship. Or, I don't do anything right, so I can't stick to healthy habits.

Sometimes the story is a trauma that happened to us - or how we were wronged by someone else. Every time we think the defeating thoughts they become more ingrained in our heads; more true, more self-defining and more destructive. What's your story?

"I was always a fat kid. My mother tortured me by putting out sweets and telling me I couldn't have them because I was fat." That's one client's story.

Write your story - or speak it into a dictation app or a text message to yourself.

Then let the story go. If you hear yourself re-telling it, tell yourself "That is no longer my story." I promise you - eventually you WILL stop hearing it.

What is your extra weight protecting you from?

Sometimes we carry extra weight as a protection from the world. Knowing what we are protecting ourselves from and allowing for that protection in other ways can break habits and patterns.

For instance, if you are a highly sensitive person and you protect yourself from the world with excess weight, you can acknowledge that and protect yourself in other ways - like taking alone time after being with groups of people.

Here are some examples of what extra weight protects us from:
- Sharing your feelings
- Being sexually attractive
- Fear of revealing your "weaknesses"
- Bullies

When you don't have the time or ability to exercise,
you can still do *this*.

Connect to your physical body.

We know that exercise makes us feel better. But it's not just the blood circulation and stretching. Connecting to our bodies enables us to tune in to what we are really feeling physically instead of what we are thinking about our bodies.

You can do this by sitting and breathing, walking, progressive relaxation (tensing and releasing your muscles from head to toe).

Physical sensations in your body at any present moment are your only reality. Your thoughts may just be an illusion that causes you to act in a way that isn't best for your body.

Tuning into your body will help you recognize the food that your body really needs to eat.

Name what you are doing

Narrating what you are doing in the present tense: folding laundry, washing dishes, driving to work, can keep you in the present moment instead of worrying about something that happened in the past or might happen in the future.

Sometimes I have been so upset about something that I have described the cars on the road to myself while driving to stop from being caught up in the upsetting thoughts or story I am telling myself.

Most of our stress comes from being in the past or the future instead of the present moment. If you can't keep yourself in the moment by narrating, try counting things, like your steps, red cars, pedestrians you pass, etc.

When we are in the present moment we are less likely to engage in emotional eating.

Write a letter to yourself
describing what your life will look like in 12 months

One of the most powerful things that I did at a point in my life when I was stuck was to write a letter to myself detailing what i wanted my life to look like in 12 months.

Almost everything that I imagined - from changes in my personal life to professional opportunities - came to be in those 12 months.

You may have heard the term "putting it out there". When we set an intention - even if we don't share it with anyone else - we are taking the first step to make a change.

If you tend to lose weight and gain it back...

Ask yourself why you feel more comfortable weighing more.

Are you worried other people will be envious?

Do you think people won't like you as a thinner person?

Do you feel uncomfortable when people ask you how much weight you've lost?

Ask yourself if those thoughts are really true.

-11-

If you self-sabotage your efforts…

What are you afraid will happen if you succeed with your weight and fitness goals?

Figure out what fear is causing you to derail your efforts.

Are you afraid of missing out on something, such as the taste of some food or the immediate gratification?

Are you afraid to disappoint someone by not eating what he or she is eating?

Are you living up to someone else's label for you?

We tend to live up to whatever label we were given in our family of origin. If we were the fat kid, the smart kid or the funny kid we tend to live up to that label.

Sometimes labels have implications - like "smart girls can't be sexy". Or, you are uncoordinated; therefore you couldn't succeed at fitness. This was very true for me. I remember when my trainer told me that he hadn't trained a woman as athletic as me since he trained a college rower. I almost fell over. I would never have considered myself athletic. I was bad at every sport I ever tried. But now that I see myself as athletic I am able to outperform my 16-year-old daughter in some aspects of fitness.

The same is true if we were labeled the picky eater. We may avoid eating vegetables to live up to that label.

What were you labeled by your family or childhood friends, and are you still living up to the label - and does that influence how you take care of your body?

Talk to yourself as if you were your own best friend

There are so many ways we can beat ourselves up with negative self-talk. We say things to ourselves we would probably never say to our best friend.

Whether it's how we look in clothing or why we are in a less than ideal work situation - the endless loop of "I can't" and "That's why I'm not ..." keeps us from succeeding even before we start.

Notice when you are engaged in negative self talk and ask yourself what you would say to your best friend if she or he were to tell you that was how she was feeling.

Put your hand on your heart when you say it. Call yourself something sweet like "honey" or "sweetheart".

Order your food to control the chaos

Many of us live with more busy stress than worry stress. We're taking care of the grandkids, their parents (our kids), spouses and pets. We're cooking, running errands, keeping kids occupied and taking them to school and activities. We are working multiple jobs and they aren't even as energy consuming as everything else. Getting on top of our food seems impossible.

But, putting our food in order can actually help control all the other chaos. When we organize what we eat, and are eating healthy food on a regular schedule, our mood is better and we can focus on keeping everything else in order.

You don't have to cook everything from scratch or prepare elaborate meals. You just have to plan ahead.

An omelet with vegetables + fruit - or - a protein smoothie = breakfast, done.

Salad + protein + roasted vegetables - or - lentil soup = lunch, done.

Protein + salad + vegetable - or - protein + vegetable + another vegetable = dinner, done.

If that doesn't float your boat, make your own meal system, shop one or two days a week and stick to it.

-15-

When eating at a restaurant, ask for what you want

Clients often tell me that eating out at restaurants derails their healthy eating. Going to a restaurant and ordering something just because it is on the menu may not be taking care of you.

You *can* ask the server for what you want. I have a client who lost a lot of weight and eliminated a lot of health problems by eating a very specific diet. She also eats out for almost every meal. But she is unwilling to eat food that gives her symptoms and causes her to gain weight. She is also unwilling to give up meals out with her family and friends.

Before she goes to a restaurant she looks at the menu ahead of time. If she doesn't see something she can work with, she calls ahead and asks if she can get something that works for her. They almost always accommodate her. She also carries her own high quality olive oil and sometimes nuts and seeds to put on a plain salad and make it filling enough to get her to the next meal.

Many of us order food we really don't want to eat to make it easier for the server, or to appear easy going to the people with whom we are eating. Ask yourself if you are more concerned with taking care of other people when you eat out than taking care of yourself. If you start taking care of yourself, you aren't difficult or annoying. You would be self-advocating for your own health and wellness.

When eating at a restaurant, order first

Clients who eat out for business meals with co-workers have told me that they are all set to order something "healthy", then someone else makes an unhealthy choice and that influences their decision - so they order something unhealthy.

Break this habit by ordering first, before another person's choice can influence you.

If appetizers are being ordered to share, and it's not something you want to eat, but you will because you are splitting the check, order a salad, or decide that your own health and wellbeing is worth more than the few dollars you will kick in for the nachos.

Think of what foods you need to eat instead of what foods you "can't" eat

Feeling deprived often keeps us from sticking to a healthy eating plan. We think about the foods we can't eat, and in some cases convince ourselves we couldn't live without them.

Instead, focus on the foods that you need to eat to feel healthy and energetic. A diet filled with the foods that make you feel good will take the emphasis off the foods that you are eliminating. You will start to look forward to eating those foods and think less and less about the others.

With many clients, adding more and more healthy foods to their diet naturally pushes out less healthy foods and before they realize it, their entire diet has changed.

This is especially true of clients who have a non-adventurous "white food" diet. Once they start experimenting with different vegetables, flavorful food preparation and good fat foods like nuts and avocados the "junk" disappears from their diet.

Bring your own food

One of the most common reasons or excuses that we use for going off of our healthy eating plan is restaurant food and social gatherings. There is an easy way to eliminate this obstacle: bring your own food.

Before you say it's rude to bring your own food to a social gathering, or not permitted to bring outside food to a restaurant, let me share my own experience. I have a daughter with severe food allergies. She can only eat food that she prepares. She never, ever eats food from a restaurant or shared food at a social gathering. She always brings her own.

Trust me, a party host would rather not worry about meeting your specific food requirements, and the needs and desires of every guest with a special diet. By bringing your own food, you relieve your own stress and the stress of those around you.

In almost 10 years of food allergy management, only 2 restaurants have objected to bringing our own food. One was a vegetarian/vegan restaurant that just wanted to make sure my daughter wasn't eating animal food in front of people who would be opposed - once we assured them her meal was indeed vegan, they were fine. The other restaurant was in a touristy area and probably wasn't focused on retaining patrons as regular customers. After realizing that they had looked really bad by refusing to accommodate someone with special food needs they gave us a gift card to come back. It is a good idea to call ahead and make sure bringing your own food is acceptable. But to a non-restaurant venue it's an easy way to be sure you can eat what you need.

Be clear on your goals

In my experience, clients who are really, really clear on their goals have the most success achieving meaningful and measurable change.

One of my clients was a woman in her 70's. She knew how many pounds she wanted to lose, what clothing she wanted to fit back into and what she wanted her waist measurement to be. In about 8 weeks she lost 15 pounds, achieved all her other goals and she was done. She said, "I am never going back to my old way of eating again!"

Her buddy, who did the program with her, had less specific goals and she had far less success.

I always encourage clients to make specific measurable goals that we can check back on as we work together. If you aren't clear on your goals, how will you ever know if you meet them?

One of my colleagues is a fitness trainer. He finds clients put out far less effort if their goals are vague – such as "improving health" vs. "lowering my blood pressure so I can go off my meds".

What's your "Why"?

If specific goals aren't your motivator - you might be motivated by a deeper reason for putting in the effort.

Preventing a disease that is common in your family or eating healthy and getting in shape in memory of a loved one may be your reason for wanting to eat healthy.

Or maybe you want to see your grandkids grow up or your kids get married. Even if your life isn't threatened, being motivated by something deeply personal and important to you will keep you on track when you don't feel like complying with your healthy eating and exercise plan. Health and fitness coaches call it the "why".

It will be the reason you get out of bed early in the morning to exercise or the reason for passing up the doughnuts in the office.

Write what's taking up too much brain space

Stress, anxiety and negative thoughts can cause us to fixate on things that may lead to unhealthy eating habits.

One way to get those thoughts out of your head is to put them on paper. Writing down what is taking up too much brain space is a good way to express and experience those thoughts and feelings and move on. I find this is especially helpful before bed. The better we sleep, the better we eat.

You could practice this when you get home from work if you do most of your stress eating in the evening. It would be a great way to download the day and create a binge-free atmosphere for the evening.

The can't-think-about-THAT-when-you-are- _____ rule

Worrying can lead to mindless eating. One trick that I use to keep worrying from impacting my sleep or eating habits are my mental rules. Basically, I can't think about my stressors when I am lying in bed - that's one rule.

My stressors may change from something going on with my daughters to a relationship I am struggling with to something related to my work. Whatever the stressors are at the moment - they are not allowed in my head when I am in my bed.

The same rule can be applied to riding in the car (where we often commit a lot of mindless eating) or cooking dinner in the kitchen (where there is a lot of food around) or hanging out in the kitchen or family room at night.

The rule technique is kind of like the directions for meditating. A thought floats by in your head while you are trying to meditate; you label it a thought and let it go. A worrying thought happens when you are in your sacred space - You label it worrying and let it go.

Improve your sleep with yoga nidra

Because eating well and sleeping well are so closely related, it's very important to get a full night's sleep.

One way to do that is with deep progressive relaxation or yoga nidra. Yoga nidra is a guided meditation that walks you through the process of relaxing your mind and your body and tapping into your body's own mechanisms to bring on sleep while you are lying in bed or trying to sleep on a plane or other place.

You can find yoga nidra recordings online. If you attend yoga classes with a teacher who does a yoga nidra at the end of class as a deep relaxation, you can ask the teacher if he or she would be okay if you used your phone to record her guidance.

I have found that if I have trouble relaxing a muscle - if I tense it and then relax it I am able to let go.

If you would like to do deep relaxation without using an audio prompt:
1. Start at the top of your head
2. Feel yourself relax your eyes into your sockets
3. Let your tongue rest in the bottom of your mouth.
4. Let there be a gap between your teeth.
5. Relax your jaw.
6. Feel as if your shoulders are melting down the back of your body.
7. Go down one side of your body and up the other relaxing every muscle in your arms, legs, abdomen and lower belly.

Be aware of negativity bias

Our brains are wired to a negativity bias. This means that we are always looking over our shoulders for tigers or some other predator ready to bring us down. It's a self-protection mechanism that has evolved over thousands of years. And it's not as helpful to us as it was to our ancient ancestors. Negative experiences are immediately imbedded in our brains. Positive experiences on the other hand take concentration to become a lasting impression. The reason for this is that this survival mechanism is located in the instinctual part of our brain. So, it's hard to turn it off.

What does this mean for our eating habits?

Negative thoughts more often lead to our self-destructive behaviors than our positive thoughts lead to self-nurturing behaviors. If someone says something that insults us or makes us feel badly, it's more likely to stick with us all day than if someone says something nice. When was the last time someone told you that you looked good and that led you to think, "And I feel so good, I think I'll have a salad for lunch instead of a burger"? It's more often that someone says something that makes us feel badly about ourselves and we give in to an unhealthy comfort food.

All those negative thoughts are there with us at the end of the day when we are battling the urge to eat the Girl Scout cookies. Or when we are thinking about making a healthy dinner, but then give up the idea to takeout or the hunk of cheese in the refrigerator.

So how do we counter this so that we don't let negative thoughts influence our food choices?
- When you repeat a negative encounter or comment to yourself - acknowledge that it was one thought, feeling or interchange - it doesn't define you. You can even ask yourself if it is really true, often it isn't.
- When you experience something positive, pause and take it in. Embed the positive feeling in your body and your mind.
- Realize that you don't have to be in survival mode.

Teach others how to support your efforts

One of my clients complained that her friends and family didn't take her food needs seriously.

She has symptoms associated with several different autoimmune diseases and avoids certain foods. The problem is that she is inconsistent and often eats her "forbidden foods" then puts up with the physical pain and other symptoms afterwards.

Her friends and family perceive that she doesn't take her food sensitivities seriously - so why should they? If you want others to be supportive of your healthy eating efforts, be consistent and show and tell them how you want to be treated.

If you have been inconsistent in the past, own it. Tell your friends and family, "I know I haven't been consistent in avoiding the foods that cause me _____ (name your symptom - for my client it was joint pain, stomach discomfort and headaches), but I am making a new effort to be totally consistent with my food needs. I would appreciate your support helping me avoid eating _____ (fill in your foods).

If you are trying to lose weight, but often give in to eating a lot of junk food and desserts - then wonder why your family doesn't take your healthy eating efforts seriously - you can also own it, express your renewed commitment and ask for help.

Look for the "shift" moment

Look for the "shift" moment. Then, take yourself back to that feeling when you feel like giving up. My clients describe it all the time. It's that moment when they start to feel so much better because they are eating healthier. Their anxiety decreases, their energy increases -- they feel lighter.

I experienced this recently when I got back to my regular exercise routine after weeks of busyness and illness. The first several days I felt like I was dragging my body through the motions. Then on the third or fourth day right in the middle of my workout my body started to feel really good.

Now, I can draw on that feeling to motivate myself to get back to it each day. We can call on the same feeling when we need to make healthy choices in the grocery store, at a restaurant or at our own refrigerator.

Disassociate comfort with food

Disassociate comfort and pleasure with food and associate it with other things. When we are out to a meal with friends or family, the pleasure is in sharing the time and experience with people we care about - not about what we are putting in our mouths.

When we are unhappy, going for a walk is a healthier pick-me-up than eating something sweet, salty or high in fat. There are many ways to improve our emotional state that don't involve eating.

Sometimes it's hard to tell when we are really hungry, or seeking an emotional pick-me-up.

Practicing what I call "the cauliflower test" can help us discern when we are really hungry or reaching for something to put us in a better mood.

Here's how it works: cut up some raw cauliflower and put it in a bowl to have handy in the refrigerator. At night (or after school or work) when you want to grab a snack ... and you're thinking, "Am I really hungry? Or, am I just bored, or in a habit of eating at this time?"
Grab the cauliflower. If you are really hungry, you'll eat the raw cauliflower. If it seems unappealing, you probably aren't hungry so explore what you really need.

Think about it, physical hunger is a lot easier to satisfy than emotional hunger. Try not to think of cravings or desire to eat sweet, salty or high fat food as being "just" an emotional craving that should be ignored because it isn't a physical need to eat.

In fact, it's almost more important to attend to a desire to fill an emotional lack with food. If you ignore a physical hunger cue you might get a headache, it will eventually pass, and mealtime will come again. But if you ignore emotional hunger it will keep resurfacing again and again until you get to the root of your need and address it.

Write your success story

If you've "fallen off the wagon" and you are looking to get back on, write out everything that you did when you were taking care of your nutrition and fitness:

- When you went grocery shopping
- When you cooked
- When you ate
- What you ate
- When you went to the gym or exercised

Use that story as your guide to getting back to your good habits.

See healthy foods as treats

We think of "treats" as foods we desire but "shouldn't" eat. Which leads to a whole push-pull relationship with food.

We think of "healthy" food as food that we "have to" eat or "should" eat but not the food we desire.

What if we stopped thinking of eating "healthy" as some sort of punishment or something to put up with and we truly desired the foods that are healthiest for our bodies?

What if veggies were the fun food to eat, and packaged foods were the punishment?

How do you already see vegetables and other "compliant" foods as your treats?

If you don't how could you change your perspective to see food this way?

De-clutter your space

Clutter causes stress and stress causes weight gain. Living in a cluttered space is time consuming and may lead to less time to prepare food, meal skipping or eating more restaurant food. It may lead to just throwing on clothes rather than thoughtful outfits that make you feel good about your body.

Cleaning up is also a physical activity that builds muscles. It's also an emotional activity. When our surroundings are neat and spacious we have room to think about how we can weed the junk out of our lives - packaged foods, screen time, bad relationships, and unwanted habits.

Making our space more livable, lovely and attractive can be an act of self-care.

Unless ...

Sometimes we can use cleaning and sorting our exterior environment as a way to avoid cleaning and sorting our personal life, career direction or relationships.

It's healthier when outer and inner clearing go hand-in-hand. And often activities like de-cluttering physical space can be contemplative and a pre-cursor to straightening out the inner mess.

But if you find yourself constantly cleaning the garage, reorganizing the basement or weeding the garden; ask yourself whether you are avoiding making a different kind of change or addressing a different kind of mess.

Unravel picky eating habits

Picky eating may be masking control issues and disordered eating. This can become an excuse for not eating healthy. Sometimes when life feels like it is out of our control, the one thing we can control is what we put in our mouths, and we can do it in a self-destructive way.

If you find yourself practicing picky eating habits that compromise your nutrition, ask yourself what is at the root of it.
- What are you gaining by your nutrition practices?
- Do you get attention for your pickiness?
- Do you have an issue with food textures? That can be tied to sensory processing issues because the mouth is the most sensitive part of the body. If you physically have trouble eating the foods that you know are good for you because of their texture, look at ways to desensitize yourself to gradually eat the difficult foods.

Do the opposite

If what you have been doing is not working for you, try doing the opposite. This can relate to what you are eating and how you are eating it.

If eating a high carb breakfast like oatmeal leaves you hungry in an hour, try eating something low carb and high protein. If eating a high protein breakfast leaves you sluggish, switch to a higher carb breakfast.

If eating dinner and reading or watching TV leaves you raiding the pantry at night, do something completely different with your routine so that you and the temptations aren't in proximity at that vulnerable time. You don't necessarily have to maintain the different behavior forever - just long enough to break the habit.

If all your social activities revolve around a bottle of wine, switch it up and start meeting your pals for a walk instead of a drink. Get creative. You might discover a new past time that you love.

Commit to a reasonable time frame

You can do anything for a month.

If you are struggling to drop a habit, commit to doing it for a relatively short period of time. Once you try another way, you may never go back.

This is a great practice to use to break a sugar habit, eliminate dairy or to start a new healthy habit like eating greens every day.

You could also use this practice to establish good self-care practices that you know will lead you to healthier eating:
- Meditation
- Journaling
- Going to sleep at a certain time
- Getting up and starting your day

Keep it simple

When you are trying to establish new healthy eating habits, don't try to incorporate a lot of changes all at the same time or try to follow a complicated plan or menu that requires hours of cooking each day.

Make changes one at a time. You'll also be able to assess which foods make you feel the best. You can be methodical, and start with breakfast and move through the day.

Eat the same basic thing each day, then once you get the hang of it, you can start swapping like items for like items to get some variety.

Eating the same basic diet is also efficient – you don't have to put a lot of thought into your food. When you're not thinking about what you are eating, you are less likely to debate options and just do it.

Write it down

I recently met with a client who had worked with a grocery store nutritionist, but had failed to really follow any eating plan she put forward. He told me he thought the plan I gave him was more doable.

When I asked him why, he told me it was because my plan was more detailed. What he really meant was that I wrote it down for him: breakfast, lunch, dinner and snacks – rather than giving him a list of foods to eat and expecting him to put them together to make meals or showing him the areas of the grocery to find healthy choices.

Once he could see the eating plan written down, he could go to the store and buy the food. Once the food was in the refrigerator he could fix it (because it was also simple meal assembly). Writing something down makes it actionable, it's not just an "idea".

You can write down your own eating plan, sleeping plan or exercise plan. You can make yourself a checklist of the number of glasses of water or cups of greens you intend to eat in a day.

Plan "X"

A lot of people profess to have healthy eating habits, yet they can't reach their goals.

Buy an inexpensive calendar and find a red and green marker, or any colors that make sense to you.

On days that you have "good" eating practices put an "x" in green. On the days that you don't stick to your eating plan put a red "x" on the calendar.

It's simple and not time consuming. It gives you a way to track yourself to see if you really are practicing your healthy habits. You may find that you have many more "red" days than "green" days. That will explain why you aren't reaching your goals. In other words, you thought you were sticking to your eating plan, but when you actually account for it, you see that you aren't.

If you know that one particular thing is sabotaging your efforts, like wine or cheese or fancy coffee drinks, use a different colored marker to indicate days you consume that food. It may be more often than you think. The accountability calendar will give you a clear picture of the changes you need to make to reach your goals.

Create a pampering presentation

We can make healthy food or a small snack feel indulgent with presentation, and where and how we choose to consume it. Feeling taken care of increases our level of satisfaction and we're less likely to go looking for more food.

Here are some examples:
- Cutting up fruit to eat with a small piece of cheese like bite-size rounds of Brie.
- Sipping herbal tea while relaxing after work, before jumping into chores and cooking dinner.
- Drinking seltzer water from a wine glass with a twist.
- Putting out small dishes of olives and nuts and berries for a snack rather than eating from containers.
- Using pretty dishes.
- Putting a few frozen berries in a bottle of water.

Buy a poor substitute for your comfort food

I owe this one to my daughter who could eat a pint of her favorite coconut ice cream in 2 sittings. She discovered if she bought a variety that doesn't taste as good as her favorite, she would eat less of it.

She can satisfy her craving but not go overboard.

Find a healthier substitute

If you have one food that is derailing your healthy eating efforts find a clean substitute that will give you the emotional feeling you get from the less healthy food.

If wine derails you, try herbal tea or sparkling water.

If it's ice cream, try pureed frozen banana.

Or as my daughter does for her ice cream habit - eat frozen berries instead.

If it's chips, bake your own chickpeas tossed with your favorite spices for a crunchy snack.

Be honest with yourself

Write down all the excuses you use for why you don't eat healthy or take care of yourself:
- Your work schedule
- Watching the grandkids
- Someone is sick
- The kids activities
- Food likes and dislikes
- What other people in your family eat
- Who does the cooking in your household
- Social obligations
- Family obligations

Acknowledge that despite all of these factors, you could put healthy food in your body.

What are you waiting for?

Write a list of all the things you perceive you will do once you lose weight, have more energy and get your eating habits under control.

Then next to each one, make a note of how you can start doing that now.

You might be putting off changing your eating habits because you are actually afraid of doing whatever that thing is.

- Go on a hiking vacation - *Start taking daily walks.*
- Join a gym - *Look for an exercise class, they are less intimidating. Recruit a friend to go with you.*
- Buy new (smaller) clothes - *Buy a few outfits that you feel great wearing. You'll feel better about your body.*

Change your schedule

If you experience out of control eating at a certain time of the day or evening, re-arrange your schedule so that you are not available to eat at that time.

For instance, if you struggle with eating after dinner, sign up for a fitness or yoga class or get in a book group or card game (not the kind that serves a lot of junk food).

Changing your schedule can take you out of your kitchen or family room at the time when you are most likely to over indulge.

Go to the library, take a walk outside or walk around the mall if you don't want to socialize or pay for a class.

One of my clients did laps walking around the inside of his garage in the winter to keep from sitting around watching TV and eating in the evening. He was able to eliminate diabetes medication and lose weight as a result!

-43-

Unplug

We eat when we are stressed or emotionally charged.

The state of affairs in our communities, countries and the world can cause a lot of anxiety, sadness and anger.

One way to keep those stressors out of our life and take care of our own emotional wellbeing is to stop reading, watching and listening to news.

They say, "Ignorance is bliss". In this case, it could be.

Double your veggies

Instead of eating a protein, a vegetable and a starch for dinner, have a protein and two vegetables. Or, eat a protein a vegetable and a salad.

Vegetables are detoxifying and have lots of fiber so they keep you full. You feel like you ate a proper meal, yet it is simple and fast to prepare. Just about any meat, fish or chicken can be cooked in 10 minutes in a cast iron skillet with some olive, grape seed or avocado oil.

Why does it matter that we feel like we ate a proper meal? If we feel dissatisfied we will go looking for more food.

Note: Corn is not a vegetable. It's a grain.

Have non-food indulgences

When we feel taken care of we don't have to put anything in our mouth to make us feel good.

It could be ...
- Playing a sport
- Taking a walk
- Listening to music
- Taking a bath
- Reading a book
- Getting a massage from a family member
- Giving yourself a manicure or pedicure
- Writing a note or letter
- Ironing your clothes so that you have beautifully pressed choices in the morning
- Lighting a candle

FOMO - Fear Of Missing Out

Fear of missing out can cause us to do things we know aren't good for our health such as: staying out late, eating out and over indulging of any kind.

We may even experience fear of missing out on a food that *might* taste great. We've all had the birthday cake that looked amazing and tasted like paste.

Ask yourself:
- What are you afraid you won't have or get?
- Will that really diminish your life?
- What is the value of having the piece of cake or glass of wine relative to feeling good in your body?
- Is your FOMO mindset keeping you out of your body and from following your body's natural cues?

Pick one thing

Trying to change all of your unwanted habits related to eating is a recipe for disaster. It's kind of like trying to run a marathon your first time back to exercising.

Pick one habit to change: either the easiest habit to change or the habit that you think will have the most profound impact on how you feel and look.

- If you eat bagels in the morning - replace them with bananas.
- If you drink wine while making dinner - replace it with seltzer or herbal tea.
- If you have dessert with dinner - have fruit
- If you put sugar in your coffee - cut it out - cold turkey

You get the idea.

Eat only when you are hungry

The diet culture has taught us to "always have healthy snacks on hand" to prevent eating the "wrong" thing and to "eat 5 small meals a day" to keep our metabolism up and our blood sugar stabilized.

The result is that many of us are afraid to feel hungry. As if hunger is a wild abandon to be avoided at all cost.

If we get hungry we might...
- Lose control
- Eat "bad" food
- Eat too much food

The truth is ... hunger is natural. Hunger is our body's cue it's time to eat. Hunger and satiety are nature's way of telling us when to eat and how much.

The trouble is - we often let our head tell us when to eat and how much to eat instead of our bellies.

Yet, if we start listening to our body's cues we would actually eat more of what our body needs when it needs it and skip food when it doesn't.

We play into the diet culture, which is a multi-billion dollar industry; by eating foods we think we "should" eat - like a salad with no protein or fat. Which causes us to feel hungry, lethargic and headache-y. The next thing we know we're at the vending machine or convenience store or coffee place.

OR

We eat 5 "small" meals or 3 meals and 2 snacks thinking that preventing our bodies from getting to a natural state of hunger will cause us to eat better. In reality, we may be consuming far more calories than we need - or eating at a time when we don't need food.

AND

In addition to the fact that this method goes against our physical human nature ... it has us thinking about food and eating all day long!!! You almost can't help but over consume when you are doing that!

Do an experiment. Let yourself eat only when you're hungry - see what happens. If you are like most of my clients you will find out what time of day YOU are hungriest. It's not the same for everyone. Then you can plan your meals around that. Make your largest meal at the hungriest time.

You will probably end up eating far less food if you follow your hunger cues.

Re-classify macronutrients

The diet culture teaches us to think about foods in categories of Carbs, Fat and Protein. I like to teach clients to think of foods in terms of Energy, Satiety and Muscle. We have too many negative connotations associated with the words "carb" and "fat". The truth is - without the complex carbs of vegetables and fruit - we would have a very poor immune system. Good fats control everything from our ability to think straight to our sex drive. And they keep us from overeating, because they create the feeling of satisfaction that helps us push away from the table.

Fruits, vegetables and whole grains give us energy.

Animal meat, eggs, dairy, tofu, beans and nuts and whole grains build and maintain muscle.

Nuts, seeds, avocado, olive and grape seed oil keep us satisfied and slow down a rise in blood sugar so that our energy lasts longer.

Find your foods

I eat almost the same thing every day, yet I eat a huge variety of food. When I stray from my usual foods or overeat something that I normally eat in moderation I can feel it. And I hate feeling badly.

One day I skipped breakfast, ate breakfast at lunchtime - my aggregate food consumption for the day was a meal down and I had a very active calorie burning morning - and I was working on a writing project that required energy. I didn't want to waste time on meal prep so I grabbed some cheese and crackers and headed to my desk. While doing my work I ate all the cheese and a good amount of crackers. I immediately felt like a needed a nap. That was an epic food fail.

Another day I came in from work hungry and went for some peanut butter because it was there, and easy to grab. The only problem is - peanut butter does NOT agree with my stomach. I spent the rest of the afternoon suffering when I could have taken 5 minutes to prepare myself my usual lunch.

When those things happen to you - what do you do?

Don't beat yourself up for making a bad choice. View the body signals as the results of an experiment. Take note of the foods that make your body feel good, and the foods that don't. If you are like me - you know which few foods to avoid. If you are like some of my clients you need to avoid a lot of foods. Whichever category you fall into, I am willing to bet there are still a lot of fruits and vegetables you can easily eat, some grains and some protein sources. Stick to your foods and you will feel better. When you feel better you can do the things you love, and chances are, if you are doing that - you aren't thinking about food at all!

AFTERWORD

The way we do one thing is the way we do anything

Hopefully you have a sense that the practices in the book could help you shift into healthier habits in just about any aspect of your life. Changing and getting clear on how we meet our body's needs for food can help us get clear on how to meet our needs for other things, like intimacy, companionship and job satisfaction.

If you found this book helpful and my approach in line with how you would like to improve your nutrition and your health, take **my free online nutrition assessment** on my website: nancypopkin.com.

If you would like to work with me, I offer one-on-one nutrition coaching where we will dive deeper into your habits with the hope of breaking them once and for all. There's more information on my website about that, too.

ACKNOWLEDGEMENTS

Thank you to my clients. I am honored that you allow me to work with you to change your habits in such a deeply personal and intimate aspect of your life.

Thank you to my daughters. Annabelle and Lily Roth you are my best teachers.

Thank you to my dear friend Rebekah Zhuraw. I will always be grateful for your support, accountability and brilliance.

Made in the USA
Middletown, DE
03 June 2018